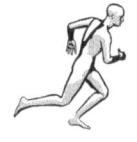 # RUN! RUN! RUN!
WORKOUT PLANNER
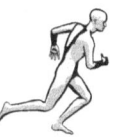

DATE:

DISTANCE	TIME	HR
DAY 1		
DAY 2		
DAY 3		
DAY 4		
DAY 5		

NOTES:

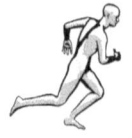 # RUN! RUN! RUN!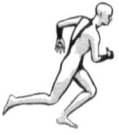
WORKOUT PLANNER

DATE:

	DISTANCE	TIME	HR
DAY 1			
DAY 2			
DAY 3			
DAY 4			
DAY 5			

NOTES:

_____

_____

_____

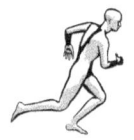 # RUN! RUN! RUN!
WORKOUT PLANNER
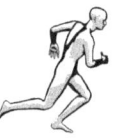

DATE:

	DISTANCE	TIME	HR
DAY 1			
DAY 2			
DAY 3			
DAY 4			
DAY 5			

NOTES:

_____

_____

_____

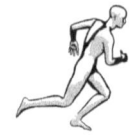 # RUN! RUN! RUN!
WORKOUT PLANNER
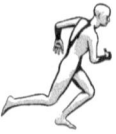

DATE:

	DISTANCE	TIME	HR
DAY 1			
DAY 2			
DAY 3			
DAY 4			
DAY 5			

NOTES:
_____
_____
_____

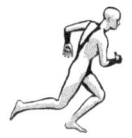 # RUN! RUN! RUN!
WORKOUT PLANNER
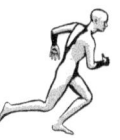

DATE:

	DISTANCE	TIME	HR
DAY 1			
DAY 2			
DAY 3			
DAY 4			
DAY 5			

NOTES:

_____

_____

_____

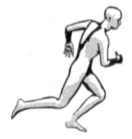 # RUN! RUN! RUN!
WORKOUT PLANNER
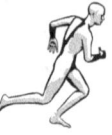

DATE:

DISTANCE	TIME	HR
DAY 1		
DAY 2		
DAY 3		
DAY 4		
DAY 5		

NOTES:

_____

_____

_____

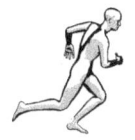 # RUN! RUN! RUN!
WORKOUT PLANNER
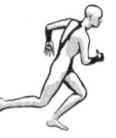

DATE:

DISTANCE	TIME	HR
DAY 1		
DAY 2		
DAY 3		
DAY 4		
DAY 5		

NOTES:

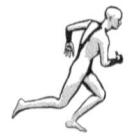 # RUN! RUN! RUN!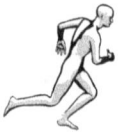
WORKOUT PLANNER

DATE:

	DISTANCE	TIME	HR
DAY 1			
DAY 2			
DAY 3			
DAY 4			
DAY 5			

NOTES:

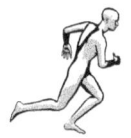 # RUN! RUN! RUN!
WORKOUT PLANNER
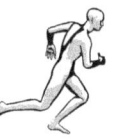

DATE:

	DISTANCE	TIME	HR
DAY 1			
DAY 2			
DAY 3			
DAY 4			
DAY 5			

NOTES:

_____

_____

_____

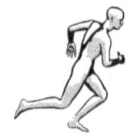 # RUN! RUN! RUN!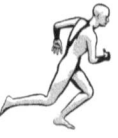
WORKOUT PLANNER

DATE:

	DISTANCE	TIME	HR
DAY 1			
DAY 2			
DAY 3			
DAY 4			
DAY 5			

NOTES:

_____

_____

_____

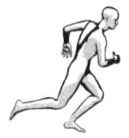 # RUN! RUN! RUN! ## WORKOUT PLANNER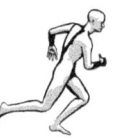

DATE:

	DISTANCE	TIME	HR
DAY 1			
DAY 2			
DAY 3			
DAY 4			
DAY 5			

NOTES:

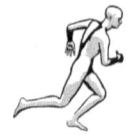 # RUN! RUN! RUN!
WORKOUT PLANNER
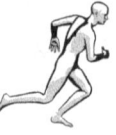

DATE:

	DISTANCE	TIME	HR
DAY 1			
DAY 2			
DAY 3			
DAY 4			
DAY 5			

NOTES:

_____

_____

_____

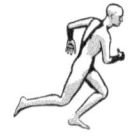 # RUN! RUN! RUN!
WORKOUT PLANNER
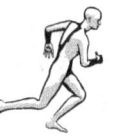

DATE:

	DISTANCE	TIME	HR
DAY 1			
DAY 2			
DAY 3			
DAY 4			
DAY 5			

NOTES:

_____

_____

_____

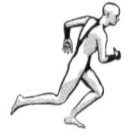 # RUN! RUN! RUN!
WORKOUT PLANNER
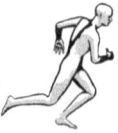

DATE:

	DISTANCE	TIME	HR
DAY 1			
DAY 2			
DAY 3			
DAY 4			
DAY 5			

NOTES:

_____

_____

_____

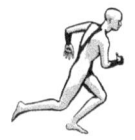 # RUN! RUN! RUN!
WORKOUT PLANNER
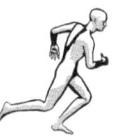

DATE:

	DISTANCE	TIME	HR
DAY 1			
DAY 2			
DAY 3			
DAY 4			
DAY 5			

NOTES:

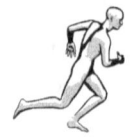 # RUN! RUN! RUN!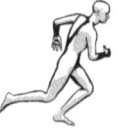
WORKOUT PLANNER

DATE:

	DISTANCE	TIME	HR
DAY 1			
DAY 2			
DAY 3			
DAY 4			
DAY 5			

NOTES:

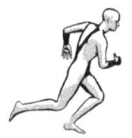 # RUN! RUN! RUN!
WORKOUT PLANNER
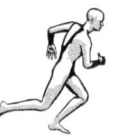

DATE:

DISTANCE	TIME	HR
DAY 1		
DAY 2		
DAY 3		
DAY 4		
DAY 5		

NOTES:

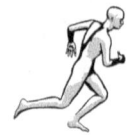 # RUN! RUN! RUN!
WORKOUT PLANNER
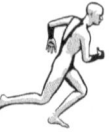

DATE:

	DISTANCE	TIME	HR
DAY 1			
DAY 2			
DAY 3			
DAY 4			
DAY 5			

NOTES:

_____

_____

_____

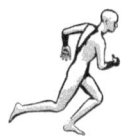 # RUN! RUN! RUN! ## WORKOUT PLANNER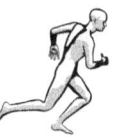

DATE:

DISTANCE	TIME	HR
DAY 1		
DAY 2		
DAY 3		
DAY 4		
DAY 5		

NOTES:

_____

_____

_____

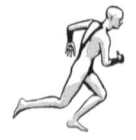 # RUN! RUN! RUN!
WORKOUT PLANNER
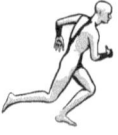

DATE:

	DISTANCE	TIME	HR
DAY 1			
DAY 2			
DAY 3			
DAY 4			
DAY 5			

NOTES:

_____

_____

_____

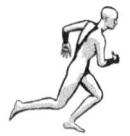 # RUN! RUN! RUN!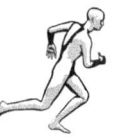
WORKOUT PLANNER

DATE:

DISTANCE	TIME	HR
DAY 1		
DAY 2		
DAY 3		
DAY 4		
DAY 5		

NOTES:

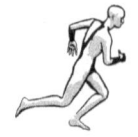 # RUN! RUN! RUN!
WORKOUT PLANNER
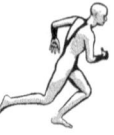

DATE:

DISTANCE	TIME	HR
DAY 1		
DAY 2		
DAY 3		
DAY 4		
DAY 5		

NOTES:

_____

_____

_____

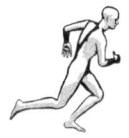 # RUN! RUN! RUN!
WORKOUT PLANNER
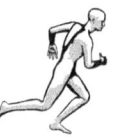

DATE:

	DISTANCE	TIME	HR
DAY 1			
DAY 2			
DAY 3			
DAY 4			
DAY 5			

NOTES:

_____

_____

_____

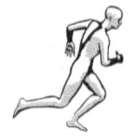 # RUN! RUN! RUN!
WORKOUT PLANNER
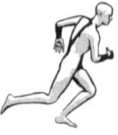

DATE:

	DISTANCE	TIME	HR
DAY 1			
DAY 2			
DAY 3			
DAY 4			
DAY 5			

NOTES:

_____

_____

_____

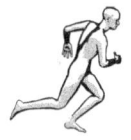 # RUN! RUN! RUN!
WORKOUT PLANNER
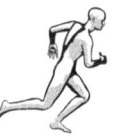

DATE:

	DISTANCE	TIME	HR
DAY 1			
DAY 2			
DAY 3			
DAY 4			
DAY 5			

NOTES:

_____

_____

_____

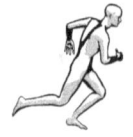 # RUN! RUN! RUN!
WORKOUT PLANNER
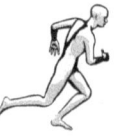

DATE:

DISTANCE	TIME	HR
DAY 1		
DAY 2		
DAY 3		
DAY 4		
DAY 5		

NOTES:

_____

_____

_____

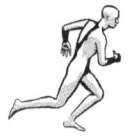 # RUN! RUN! RUN!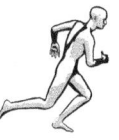
WORKOUT PLANNER

DATE:

	DISTANCE	TIME	HR
DAY 1			
DAY 2			
DAY 3			
DAY 4			
DAY 5			

NOTES:

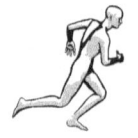 # RUN! RUN! RUN!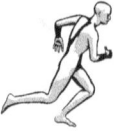
WORKOUT PLANNER

DATE:

	DISTANCE	TIME	HR
DAY 1			
DAY 2			
DAY 3			
DAY 4			
DAY 5			

NOTES:

_____

_____

_____

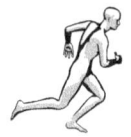 # RUN! RUN! RUN!
WORKOUT PLANNER
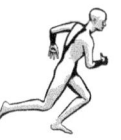

DATE:

	DISTANCE	TIME	HR
DAY 1			
DAY 2			
DAY 3			
DAY 4			
DAY 5			

NOTES:

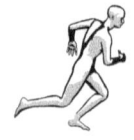 # RUN! RUN! RUN!
WORKOUT PLANNER
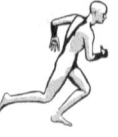

DATE:

	DISTANCE	TIME	HR
DAY 1			
DAY 2			
DAY 3			
DAY 4			
DAY 5			

NOTES:

_____

_____

_____

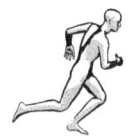 # RUN! RUN! RUN! ## WORKOUT PLANNER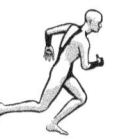

DATE:

DISTANCE	TIME	HR
DAY 1		
DAY 2		
DAY 3		
DAY 4		
DAY 5		

NOTES:

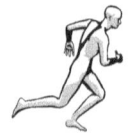 # RUN! RUN! RUN!
WORKOUT PLANNER
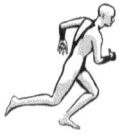

DATE:

DISTANCE	TIME	HR
DAY 1		
DAY 2		
DAY 3		
DAY 4		
DAY 5		

NOTES:

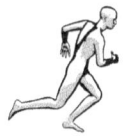 # RUN! RUN! RUN!
WORKOUT PLANNER
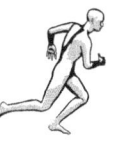

DATE:

	DISTANCE	TIME	HR
DAY 1			
DAY 2			
DAY 3			
DAY 4			
DAY 5			

NOTES:

_____

_____

_____

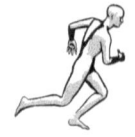 # RUN! RUN! RUN!
WORKOUT PLANNER
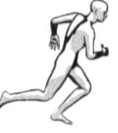

DATE:

	DISTANCE	TIME	HR
DAY 1			
DAY 2			
DAY 3			
DAY 4			
DAY 5			

NOTES:

_____

_____

_____

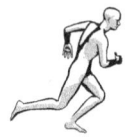 # RUN! RUN! RUN!
WORKOUT PLANNER
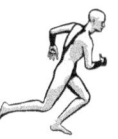

DATE:

DISTANCE	TIME	HR
DAY 1		
DAY 2		
DAY 3		
DAY 4		
DAY 5		

NOTES:

_____

_____

_____

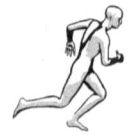 # RUN! RUN! RUN!
WORKOUT PLANNER
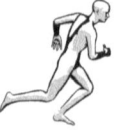

DATE:

	DISTANCE	TIME	HR
DAY 1			
DAY 2			
DAY 3			
DAY 4			
DAY 5			

NOTES:

_____

_____

_____

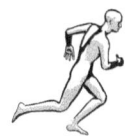 # RUN! RUN! RUN!
WORKOUT PLANNER
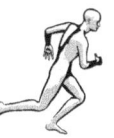

DATE:

DISTANCE	TIME	HR
DAY 1		
DAY 2		
DAY 3		
DAY 4		
DAY 5		

NOTES:

_____

_____

_____

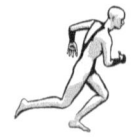 # RUN! RUN! RUN!
WORKOUT PLANNER
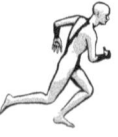

DATE:

DISTANCE	TIME	HR
DAY 1		
DAY 2		
DAY 3		
DAY 4		
DAY 5		

NOTES:

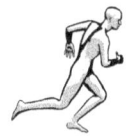 # RUN! RUN! RUN! ## WORKOUT PLANNER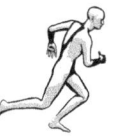

DATE:

DISTANCE	TIME	HR
DAY 1		
DAY 2		
DAY 3		
DAY 4		
DAY 5		

NOTES:

_____

_____

_____

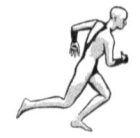 # RUN! RUN! RUN!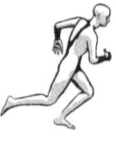
WORKOUT PLANNER

DATE:

	DISTANCE	TIME	HR
DAY 1			
DAY 2			
DAY 3			
DAY 4			
DAY 5			

NOTES:

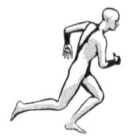 # RUN! RUN! RUN!
WORKOUT PLANNER
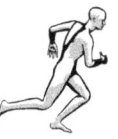

DATE:

	DISTANCE	TIME	HR
DAY 1			
DAY 2			
DAY 3			
DAY 4			
DAY 5			

NOTES:

_____

_____

_____

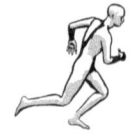 # RUN! RUN! RUN!
WORKOUT PLANNER
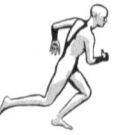

DATE:

	DISTANCE	TIME	HR
DAY 1			
DAY 2			
DAY 3			
DAY 4			
DAY 5			

NOTES:

_____

_____

_____

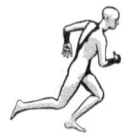 # RUN! RUN! RUN!
WORKOUT PLANNER
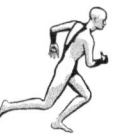

DATE:

	DISTANCE	TIME	HR
DAY 1			
DAY 2			
DAY 3			
DAY 4			
DAY 5			

NOTES:

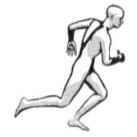 # RUN! RUN! RUN!
WORKOUT PLANNER
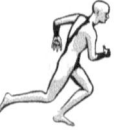

DATE:

	DISTANCE	TIME	HR
DAY 1			
DAY 2			
DAY 3			
DAY 4			
DAY 5			

NOTES:

_____

_____

_____

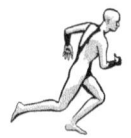 # RUN! RUN! RUN!
WORKOUT PLANNER
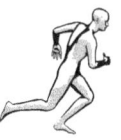

DATE:

	DISTANCE	TIME	HR
DAY 1			
DAY 2			
DAY 3			
DAY 4			
DAY 5			

NOTES:

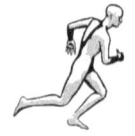 # RUN! RUN! RUN!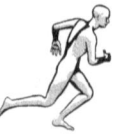
WORKOUT PLANNER

DATE:

DISTANCE	TIME	HR
DAY 1		
DAY 2		
DAY 3		
DAY 4		
DAY 5		

NOTES:

_____

_____

_____

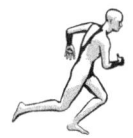 # RUN! RUN! RUN! ## WORKOUT PLANNER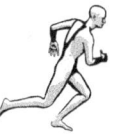

DATE:

	DISTANCE	TIME	HR
DAY 1			
DAY 2			
DAY 3			
DAY 4			
DAY 5			

NOTES:

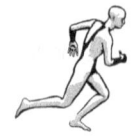 # RUN! RUN! RUN!
WORKOUT PLANNER
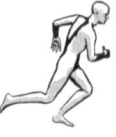

DATE:

	DISTANCE	TIME	HR
DAY 1			
DAY 2			
DAY 3			
DAY 4			
DAY 5			

NOTES:

_____

_____

_____

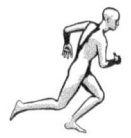 # RUN! RUN! RUN!
WORKOUT PLANNER
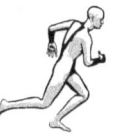

DATE:

	DISTANCE	TIME	HR
DAY 1			
DAY 2			
DAY 3			
DAY 4			
DAY 5			

NOTES:

_____

_____

_____

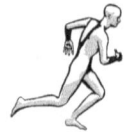 # RUN! RUN! RUN!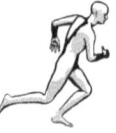
WORKOUT PLANNER

DATE:

	DISTANCE	TIME	HR
DAY 1			
DAY 2			
DAY 3			
DAY 4			
DAY 5			

NOTES:

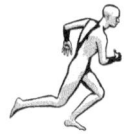 # RUN! RUN! RUN!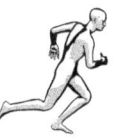
WORKOUT PLANNER

DATE:

	DISTANCE	TIME	HR
DAY 1			
DAY 2			
DAY 3			
DAY 4			
DAY 5			

NOTES:

_____

_____

_____

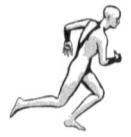 # RUN! RUN! RUN!
WORKOUT PLANNER
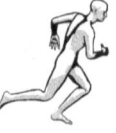

DATE:

DISTANCE	TIME	HR
DAY 1		
DAY 2		
DAY 3		
DAY 4		
DAY 5		

NOTES:

_____

_____

_____

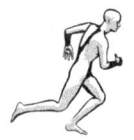 # RUN! RUN! RUN!
WORKOUT PLANNER
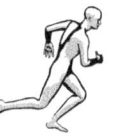

DATE:

	DISTANCE	TIME	HR
DAY 1			
DAY 2			
DAY 3			
DAY 4			
DAY 5			

NOTES:

_____

_____

_____

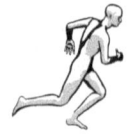 # RUN! RUN! RUN!
WORKOUT PLANNER
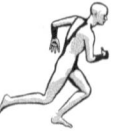

DATE:

	DISTANCE	TIME	HR
DAY 1			
DAY 2			
DAY 3			
DAY 4			
DAY 5			

NOTES:

_____

_____

_____

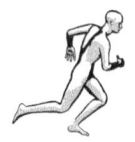 # RUN! RUN! RUN!
WORKOUT PLANNER
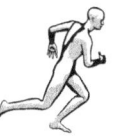

DATE:

	DISTANCE	TIME	HR
DAY 1			
DAY 2			
DAY 3			
DAY 4			
DAY 5			

NOTES:

_____

_____

_____

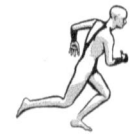 # RUN! RUN! RUN! ## WORKOUT PLANNER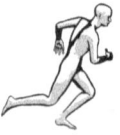

DATE:

	DISTANCE	TIME	HR
DAY 1			
DAY 2			
DAY 3			
DAY 4			
DAY 5			

NOTES:

_____

_____

_____

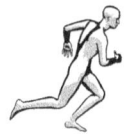 # RUN! RUN! RUN!
WORKOUT PLANNER
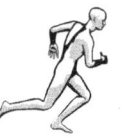

DATE:

DISTANCE	TIME	HR
DAY 1		
DAY 2		
DAY 3		
DAY 4		
DAY 5		

NOTES:

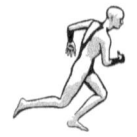 # RUN! RUN! RUN!
WORKOUT PLANNER
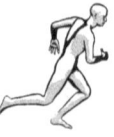

DATE:

	DISTANCE	TIME	HR
DAY 1			
DAY 2			
DAY 3			
DAY 4			
DAY 5			

NOTES:

_____

_____

_____

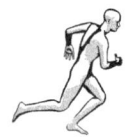 # RUN! RUN! RUN!
WORKOUT PLANNER
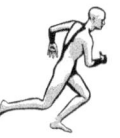

DATE:

	DISTANCE	TIME	HR
DAY 1			
DAY 2			
DAY 3			
DAY 4			
DAY 5			

NOTES:

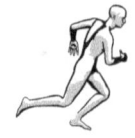 # RUN! RUN! RUN!
WORKOUT PLANNER
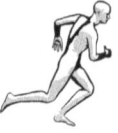

DATE:

	DISTANCE	TIME	HR
DAY 1			
DAY 2			
DAY 3			
DAY 4			
DAY 5			

NOTES:
_____
_____
_____

www.ingramcontent.com/pod-product-compliance
Lightning Source LLC
Chambersburg PA
CBHW072118280526
45788CB00006B/2540